I0438555

Best Clinical Guide for Your Family and Your Doctor

The Helper in Critical Health Situations

Onyechela Ogbonna

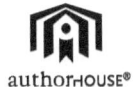

authorHOUSE®

AuthorHouse™
1663 Liberty Drive
Bloomington, IN 47403
www.authorhouse.com
Phone: 1-800-839-8640

Published by AuthorHouse 4/19/2012

ISBN: 978-1-4685-8807-1 (sc)
ISBN: 978-1-4685-8806-4 (e)

Library of Congress Control Number: 2012906961

CONTENTS

Introduction

This is a quick guide to help for medical and non-medical personnel at the point of need in hospitals, clinics, and home settings. It has clinical case scenarios, questions, and answers.

It includes a plan of action based on differential diagnoses at the point of need to help guide you during critical moments.

This powerful medical reference note reminds doctors of the different diagnoses to consider and a plan for acute situations when a life is danger or the doctor is alone. When it is nighttime and there are no support specialists, or there is no time to open a large medical book or search the Internet, he still needs to act to save a life.

This family health protection guide teaches how to understand when our beloved spouse, grandparents, children, or friends are not feeling well and how we can help them. It explains the causes of common health problems such as chest pain, headaches, slurred speech, and difficulty breathing. It offers helpful lifesaving actions.

The book encourages healthy living advice, such as regular exercise, healthy diet, alcohol and smoking cessation, age appropriate vaccinations, mammograms, and other important health topics.

Clinical Scenario One

Mr. A. is a forty-five-year-old male. He was brought to the emergency department of the community hospital after his wife called 911. His hands and legs had been shaking, and he was not responding to verbal commands.

When the emergency team arrived, they confirmed he was having seizure. He was given intravenous Ativan by the team. He has a history of heavy alcohol use. He drinks beer and vodka. He has been abusing alcohol most of his life.

His wife said that he had not had alcohol for two days because he was trying to stop drinking. He had lost his job recently due to alcohol use. He had been reporting late to work.

On physical examination in the emergency department, he has tachycardia (irregular heartbeat) and diaphoresis (excessive sweating). His face was flushed. He was awake but confused. He was hallucinating, seeing spiders and objects. He had tremors of both upper extremities.

What should you do?

A. He is withdrawing from alcohol. He needs to be admitted to the hospital for intravenous Ativan, thiamine, and alcohol withdrawal protocol. He is sick.

B.   He is malingering (intentional deceptive behavior). It is not a medical problem.

C.   He has alcohol withdrawal. He needs to resume alcohol use immediately.

The correct answer is A. He has alcohol withdrawal signs. This is a serious medical condition. He should be admitted to the hospital for treatment.

Options A and C are wrong. He tried to quit, but he needs help to do it safely because his body is addicted and dependent on alcohol. It is safe to get treatment in the hospital. Resuming his alcohol use will result in more harm. It is unsafe to leave the hospital in his current medical condition.

Alcohol and Drugs: Family Health Guide

Drugs and alcohol are very addictive and difficult to quit. The safest approach is not to start using then. If they already have their grip on you, your best option is to make every effort to quit. Drugs and alcohol damage your brain.

They also cause injuries to the liver, which is an organ needed to remove waste products from your body. Toxins will accumulate and make you sick and confused.

People who become confused due to alcohol use or drug dependence cannot function well at work or at home. The consequences include job losses and broken homes.

Drug and alcohol use are serious financial burdens to you, your family, and society in general. The financial implications are exorbitant; they come from the direct cost of obtaining drugs. People who abuse alcohol are more likely to be jobless and homeless. Society pays a big price to treat dependence-related issues that sometimes require multiple admissions to hospitals.

Healthy Habits: Regular Exercise and a Healthy Diet

Exercise regularly—outside in the fresh air if the weather permits. A simple way is to park your car at home and walk to the grocery store instead of driving. Consider getting off the bus one stop ahead and walking home.

Dancing is great exercise for your body. Switch on your favorite music and dance. It is even better when you dance with your spouse. This is not only exercise; it helps build a common interest.

Running, bicycle riding, and jogging are wonderful for healthier, younger people. Participating in gym programs with treadmills and weights can be great for those who can afford it. Alternatives include simple home exercises: pushups, stretching, or walking for thirty minutes each day. Do whatever works for your family and job schedule.

Always observe safety precautions during exercise to prevent injuries and falls. Examples of safety measures include wearing helmets when riding and avoiding wet floors. Frail people and the elderly need extra support to prevent falls and injuries.

Common Critical Hospital Situations for Medical Personnel

You are a physician on call for a local hospital in the open intensive care unit. You are on call for the entire hospital, including the ICU.

The nurse calls your direct phone because of a critical situation. She is up to date with her ACLS certifications. She has great clinical skills and more than twenty-five years of experience in the intensive care unit.

She tells you that the patient in ICU is not doing well. He is not responding to any stimuli—not even a sternal rub. There is no palpable pulse. His blood pressure cannot be recorded because it is too low. The patient is a fifty-five year old male with diabetes mellitus. He had been admitted the night before with acute renal failure and hyperkalemia (high potassium levels in the blood). He is awaiting hemodialysis. His renal has been consulted.

The nurse and her ICU colleagues have initiated ACLS protocol with good CPR. The monitor shows normal sinus rhythm. You confirm that the patient has no pulse.

The printed 12-lead electrocardiogram is normal, but the patient is unresponsive and has no pulse.

What do you call this condition?

A.   A: Sleeping Syndrome

B.   Ventricular Tachycardia

C.   Pulseless Electrical Activity

The correct answer is C. Pulseless Electrical Activity is a serious medical condition managed as per ACLS protocol. This is a life-threatening condition. When in doubt, call senior doctors.

Option A is wrong because he is not sleeping. He is dying. Act immediately.

Option B is wrong. Ventricular Tachycardia is different because the electrocardiogram will appear ugly—not normal.

Family Health Guide: Why Are All These Wires and Machines Connected To Me?

Many patients admitted to the hospital with serious conditions are connected to wires called cardiac monitors. They are used to continuously monitor the heart for abnormal rhythms, which is when the heart starts working in abnormal state. It kills people if it is not identified in time.

You are a first-year medical intern excited about your first overnight call after all the effort to get into medical residency. The nurse calls and says, "Doctor, please help. The patient is not responding. I cannot feel a pulse." You hear panic, commotion and crying in the background.

What should you do?

A. Wait until you consult your senior doctors. Present the case to them and review your ACLS manual before calling the nurse back.

B. Tell the nurse to do ABCs (airways, breathing, circulation). Initiate CPR if there is no pulse as you rush to help the patient.

C.   Tell the nurse to allow the patient to sleep. He must be very tired.

The correct answer is B.

Option A and B are wrong because they will delay care for a patient in critical condition.

Remember that hospital nurse is ACLS trained. Tell her to do ABCs as you rush toward the patient to his save life. This is serious.

Remember that most hospitals have rapid response teams. Bring the crash cart and initiate ABC. Check for a pulse and start CPR immediately.

As you rush toward the patient, think of possible causes (see examples below).

Differential diagnoses include:

- Intracranial Hemorrhage. Do not forget to look for dilated pupils. The head CT will tell you when the patient is stable.
- Ventricular Tachycardia. Is the patient on a monitor? VT is a shockable rhythm.
- Myocardiac Infarction. Was the patient having chest pain or dyspnea before?
- Complete Heart Block (EKG needs to be done)
- Other Arrhythmia
- Pulmonary Emboli (any history of DVT)
- Aortic Dissection. This kills patients if missed.
- Pneumothorax. Is the breathing equal and tympanic?

- Drug Overdose. Was the patient given too much opioid because of severe pain?
- Electrolyte Abnormality. The arterial blood gas and chemistry panel will help you.

Action Plan

Remember to consult experienced doctors and nurses, but do not to delay patient care. See the doctor's menu and select which is applicable based on the specific case scenario:
- Investigations: Use updated ACLS guidelines. Focused exam, ABCD, intubation, shocks, vitals, physical examination monitors, electrocardiogram, laboratory investigations, arterial blood gas, complete blood count, chemistry panel, cardiac enzymes imaging, X-rays, and head CT.
- Medications: Ask yourself when to give any life-saving medication: aspirin, betablock, and anticoagulation during myocardial infarction. If the patient is bleeding, is there contraindication (aspirin and heparin, for example).
- Quick chart review of documentation will tell you about allergies.
- Level of care: Remember that most medical floors do not have enough staff to manage very sick patients that require too much attention. Transfer to step down or intensive care for high care after a near-death situation.
- Advanced care may be necessary in special situations: chest decompression for

pneumothorax, cardiac pacing for heart block, TPA for acute stroke, or urgent cardiac catherization for ST-elevated myocardiac infarction.

Healthy Diet: Family Health Guide

The idea of a healthy diet varies due to cultural, religious, and individual preferences. The simple rule is that a diet rich in fruit and vegetables is always great choice because it provides fiber, vitamins, and less fat. It also has high water and nutritional contents.

A high-calorie diet and fried food soaked in oil are is more likely to result in weight gain and obesity

Chest Pain: Is He Having a Heart Attack? How Can I Help?

The causes of chest pain include heart attacks, blood clots on the lungs or blood system, blood vessel rupture, chest infection, heartburn, chest trauma, and many more. Physicians are in a better position to diagnose it with modern equipment.

Mr. H. is a sixty-two-year-old male with a history of hypertension, hyperlipidemia, and coronary artery disease. He had cardiac bypass operation two years earlier after a stress test result showed three-vessel disease.

He says the chest pressure feels like an elephant is sitting on his chest. He appears sweaty and anxious. He has been holding his chest for more than forty-five minutes, but it is not resolving. He took baby aspirin without any benefit.

What should he do?

A.   Take his anti-anxiety medication and relax because he looks anxious.

B.   Call 911 and get to the emergency department right away because he might be having a heart attack.

C. Take his wife's stronger pain medication (Percocet), which her doctor prescribed for pain after her knee replacement.

The correct answer is B. Call 911 and get to the emergency department. He may be having a heart attack because chest pressure is a typical symptom for a heart attack. He has risk factors for heart attack: age, history of coronary artery disease, and a cardiac bypass operation.

Tell the nurse get an electrocardiogram on the patient. See the patient immediately and review the electrocardiogram.

If it is not myocardial infarction, what can it be? Make a mental list of possible causes:

- Myocardial Infarction. If there is STEMI on the EKG, the patient needs urgent cardiac catheterization or thrombolysis if cath lab is very far.
- Pulmonary Emboli. Patients with DVT, low INR, and limited mobility are prone to PE.
- Pericarditis. EKG of pericarditis may appear like STEMI—watch out!
- Pneumothorax. A large pneumothorax causes cardiac arrest. Check lung for equal breathing sounds. Do a portable chest X-ray.
- Aortic Dissection. A leaking large blood vessel is deadly. If this suspected, get CT angiogram.
- Pneumonia.
- GERD
- Anxiety
- Musculoskeletal

Action Plan

Perform a focused physical examination. Perform and review an electrocardiogram and compare with an old one if available. If there is an elevated ST, this is STEMI until proven otherwise. Timely intervention is crucial during myocardial infarction. Call the on-call cardiologist. Fax the electrocardiogram to him. Some hospitals have a myocardial infarction code. Get the help of more experienced doctors.

Place the patient on a cardiac monitor because arrhythmia is more likely to occur during a heart attack. Obtain a laboratory test, including cardiac enzymes to identify an enzyme leak. Use the chemistry panel. The chest X-ray may show pneumothorax as the cause of chest pain.

Think of any medication you need to give right away. Consider the patient's contraindications for any medications you need to give, such as allergies, bradycardia, or hypotension.

For MI, always review the most recent management guidelines as they change often. Recommended medications include betablocker, aspirin, plavix, nitrate, anticoagulation, ACEI, and statins. BP control to reduce demand ischemia.

If you suspect gastritis as the cause, try proton pump inhibitors such as omeprazole.

When you suspect pulmonary emboli or aortic, have a CT angiogram to rule them out.

Diffuse crackle on a physical lung physical examination may be a clue to pulmonary edema. A portable chest X-ray will you a quick answer. Intravenous furosemide will provide immediate relief for most patients. Antibiotics will be the proper treatment for pneumonia on a chest

X-ray. Do not be a medical hero; when in doubt, call the senior doctors for help.

Ms D is a fifty-year-old female. She went to her primary care physician and complained of severe shortness of acute onset a day earlier. It woke her up after she returned from vacation. The flight was thirteen hours with a two-hour stopover.

Her medical problem is diet-controlled hypertension and rheumatoid arthritis controlled on prednisone, which she takes regularly. She had a normal stress test, electrocardiogram, and echocardiogram two months earlier. She has no allergies.

The system review was unremarkable except that she noticed that her left leg had been getting bigger since yesterday. She thinks it is due to her leg position on the plane.

During the physical examination, her vitals, temperature, and blood pressure are normal. Her respiratory rate is twenty-eight per minute. Oxygen saturation on room air is 86 percent.

She appears to be in moderate respiratory distress, but she is able to complete sentences.

The lung examination is normal—no crackles. The cardiac examination is remarkable for only mild tachycardia. There is no jugular vein distension on her neck. Her left leg is obviously swollen compared to right, but it is not warm to the touch.

The chest radiograph is normal. The chemistry panel and complete blood count are normal. Her D-dimer is above 2000.

What is the most likely diagnosis and next plan?

A. She has fracture of left tibia. Do not worry about high D-dimer; it is nonspecific. Get left lower extremity radiology.

B. She has deep vein thrombosis and possible pulmonary emboli. Get pulmonary angiogram and Doppler ultrasound on her left leg.

C. She is too young to have all these problems based on what she read on the Internet. Allow her to go home. She needs to resume duty today after her vacation.

The correct answer is **B**. Use of steroids is a risk factor for deep vein thrombosis and pulmonary emboli. High D-dimer. There might be hypoxia with normal lung examination and chest X-ray. Her swollen left leg is very suspicious of a blood clot.

Options A and C are incorrect. Please ask your doctor for an explanation. This will break the ice to talk with him or other colleagues.

Warning Signs of a Serious Medical Problem

A common headache can be a sign of stroke, bleeding into the brain, a brain tumor, or other serious medical conditions. Never ignore a severe headache, headache with fever, headache with slurred speech, headache with arm or leg heaviness or weakness, headache with nausea and vomiting, headache with dizziness, headache with passing out, or headache with shaking. When in doubt, ask your doctor or call 911 if in USA.

Nurse J is a nurse in general medical floor. She has good clinical experience in neurology examination. She has worked in the neurology unit for many years.

Patient S. is a seventy-five-year-old female with a history of hypertension, carotid stenosis, hyperlipidemia, and atrial fibrillation. She is not on Coumadin yet. She has not yet decided to take it because she likes green vegetables.

She was admitted with fever and chills. She has a urinary tract infection. She is on intravenous antibiotic. She is doing well and has no more fever.

The doctor is planning to discharge her in the morning.

She calls for help at 8:30 p.m. to use the bathroom.

She is hooked up to the infusion pump for intravenous antibiotics. Nurse J goes in to help her. Patient P is very independent; she walked to the bathroom holding the infusion pump. The nurse just stood near as required by hospital policy to prevent a fall.

Patient P used the bathroom, returned to her bed without any help, and thanked Nurse J for coming to help.

Patient P needed some ice chips to wet her dry mouth. She was neurologically intact. She spoke clearly to the nurse when requesting ice chips by 8:35. She has developed slurred speech, cannot hold the ice chips with her right hand, and is falling when she tries to stand because she cannot support herself due to right leg weakness. She is drooling, her face looks different, and she has a headache.

What should the nurse do?

A. Give her the ice chips and her dinner. She will be fine.

B. Call the doctor immediately and activate the stroke team because she may be having a stroke.

C. Give her sleeping medication because she said earlier that she needs something to help her sleep.

The correct answer is B. Call the doctor and stroke team. She has acute symptoms of stroke, and she needs urgent evaluation. She may benefit from TPA because she was normal five minutes earlier.

Option A and C are wrong because they will result

in delayed care and possible aspiration pneumonitis. She should have nothing by mouth at this critical moment.

Stroke risk factors include:

- Atrial Fibrillation
- Uncontrolled Hypertension
- Cardiac Embolism
- Carotid Stenosis
- Vasculitis
- Systemic Lupus Erythromatosis
- Syphilis
- Cocaine Use

Action Plan

Many hospitals have a code stroke or stroke alert. Call them and consult neurology immediately. Protect the patient's airways. Do ABCDs and frequent neurological checks. Do not give anything by mouth during an acute stroke to prevent aspiration and more complications.

Make sure the patient's vitals are stable enough before sending for head imaging. It is not good when a patient crashes during imaging in the radiology department. It is difficult to run code blue or perform CPR in the radiology machine.

When the patient is stabilized and airways are protected, most doctors order head imaging with head CT without contrast. It is quick and informative and has few contraindications. If the head CT is negative, remember that the brain MRI is more sensitive if the patient has no contraindication. Some metal implants are incompatible with an MRI.

The use of a medication called TPA is lifesaving in some patients with acute stroke, but it has very strict conditions that need to be met before use.

You can help by documenting properly the last time the patient was found normal. The longer the time, the less likely the benefit.

Note that the guidelines and the contraindications to use TPA keep changing as more clinical research date accumulates. Please consult a neurologist to help you. When in doubt, call 911.

Why Your Doctor Says to Stop Using Tobacco

Tobacco use is not good for your health—period.

Tobacco use causes lung cancer, and worsens chronic lung disease such as Chronic Obstructive Pulmonary Disease (COPD) and asthma. It makes you more likely to have stroke or a heart attack due to changes in the blood vessels.

It is better to not start smoking—no matter how appealing it is presented to you by your best friend, role model, or advertisements. Make efforts to quit if are already smoking. Your doctor will be happy to provide you with several options to stop smoking, such as the nicotine patch.

Mr. P is a dedicated physician's assistant in the emergency department. His patient is a forty-year-old man with a history of seizures. He is not compliant with his medications because they make him feel sleepy at work.

He is presented for evaluation for a superficial laceration on his right forearm. It happened about an hour ago at work. His vaccinations are up to date, including a tetanus vaccination less than two years ago. There is no incidence of tetanus in the community.

During history and Physical, he suddenly falls on the ground, shaking his hands and legs with tonic-clonic rhythm. He foamed at the mouth, bit his tongue, and had urinary incontinence.

What is the most likely diagnosis?

A. Confusion or some psychiatric disorder

B. Hypoxia

C. Seizure

The correct answer is **C**. Tonic-clonic movement is a typical sign of a seizure. Remember that he has not been taking his seizure medication.

Tetanus needs more than an hour to develop. He has been vaccinated against tetanus, and the community has no cases of tetanus.

Hypoxia is less likely to develop suddenly with respiratory problems in a young man.

These are warning signs of serious medical problem. You can call the doctor because someone does not look good.

Elderly patients and kids may not be able to explain how they feel. Do not worry about what to tell the doctor—physicians will understand what you mean. *Grandpa does not look good. He is not eating. He is falling often. He appears lethargic. He seems confused. The baby is not her usual self. She is not playing. She is very irritable.*

Mr. C. is a sixty-five-year-old man without any medical problem. He has been living a healthy and active life. He goes to gym regularly, runs on the treadmill for hours, and eats healthily. He has no alcohol, tobacco, or drug abuse. He is not obese. He has not seen a physician for forty years because he feels great. He has never had a colonoscopy.

Recently he has been feeling very tired easily. He cannot even walk on treadmill for ten minutes. He has been losing weight unintentionally—despite a good appetite and a healthy diet. He sometimes sees blood clots in his stool after a bowel movement.

What should he do?

A. Do not worry. It will resolve with time.

B. See a doctor right away. He may have colon cancer.

C. Try natural remedies advertised on the Internet.

The correct answer is B. Unintentional weight loss and bloody stool are signs of possible colon cancer in a patient who has not had a colonoscopy.

Option A and C are wrong because they will result in delayed diagnosis and more complications. Option A is wrong because it will result to delay in proper care. A heart attack makes patient appear anxious. It is better to treat a life-threatening condition before focusing on anxiety.

Option C is wrong. It is not a good idea to use other patients' medications—no matter how close. This option will also result in delayed treatment and complications.

Warning Signs of Serious Medical Problems

Grandma feels very warm when I touch her, and she is not responding to me. These signs could be evidence of infection in the lung, pneumonia, urinary tract infection, anemia, or other serious medical problems. When in doubt, ask your doctor or call 911.

My belly hurts badly. I cannot keep food down. I have persistent diarrhea or bloody stool. Patients on Coumadin, Pradaxa, aspirin, Plavix, and ibuprofen are more likely to bleed massively. Do not wait until you are dehydrated or complications develop. Just call for help; the emergency department physician has the answer.

Difficulty breathing after minimal exertion or at rest is a serious condition. Causes include weak heart, possible heart attack, asthma attack, COPD, anemia, and a blood clot on the lung. Just tell the doctor you cannot breathe and let him figure it out.

Ms V. is a visiting nurse who just arrived to evaluate Mr. C. He is a seventy-five-year-old male with a history of smoking for over forty years. He used to smoke two packs per day, but he recently reduced it to one cigarette per day because his doctor has been encouraging him to quit.

He usually walks his dog every day. On this day, he

is not feeling well and is having difficulty breathing. He looks very sick and is using every muscle to breathe. Mrs. V. counted his respiratory rate at thirty-two per minute. He has no fever. His temperature is 97.6. She listened to his chest with her stethoscope and heard diffused expiratory wheeze and no crackle.

She called 911 and took him to the emergency department. The physician confirmed the expiratory wheeze and no crackles. His chest X-ray showed a hyper-distended lung without opacity. He responded well to the breathing treatment with nebulization albuterol and ipratropium bromide and an intravenous steroid.

What is the most likely diagnosis?

A. Chronic Obstructive Pulmonary Disease

B. Pneumonia

C. Anxiety attack

The correct answer is **A**. Smoking is a risk factor for COPD. Wheezing and a clinical response to breathing treatment are very suggestive of COPD.

Option B is incorrect. The typical clinical features of pneumonia include fever and cough. In a lung examination, you hear crackle instead of wheezing.

Option C is incorrect. An anxiety attack usually will not cause wheezing. Patients with COPD may have:

- Anxiety
- Shortness of Breath
- Difficulty Breathing

It has large differential diagnosis. Causes include:

- Asthma
- Chronic Obstructive Lung Disease
- Pneumonia
- Pulmonary Edema
- Congestive Heart Failure
- Pneumothorax
- Pulmonary Embolus
- Sepsis
- Anemia
- Anxiety
- Metabolic Acidosis
- Pleural Effusion
- Respiratory Muscle Weakness
- Obesity
- Panic Attacks
- Upper Airway Obstruction
- Restrictive Lung Disease
- Interstitial Lung
- Pleural Thickening
- Aspiration Pneumonitis
- Myocardial Ischemia
- Valvular Obstruction
- Arrhythmia
- Cardiac Tamponade
- Hypercapnia

Action Plan

- Protect Airways
- Monitor Oxygen Saturation

- Check Code Status To Prevent Intubation of Patient with DNR Status
- Examine Lung Crackle and Wheezing
- Hyperresonance
- JVD
- Evaluate Mental State

When a patient has hypoxia and shortness of breath, but the physical examination is unremarkable—and there are no crackles or wheezing—think of pulmonary emboli, especially in patients who have limited mobility, had recent surgery, leg swelling, or calf tenderness.

Please do not press the swollen calf; controversy exists that it may dislodge deep thrombosis and cause pulmonary emboli. The CT angiogram will answer the question if there are no contraindications, such as abnormal kidney function or contrast allergy.

Investigations: High yield test include chest X-ray may show pulmonary edema and arterial blood gas (may show respiratory acidosis, which will require transfer to intensive care unit or acute endotrcheal intubation or non-invasive ventilation.

Depending on the case scenario, the chemistry panel may suggest severe abnormalities. The electrocardiogram may surprise you with acute myocardial infarction. A complete blood count may tell your patient has severe anemia. Other investigations include cardiac enzymes and echocardiograms. When in doubt, please call 911. Consider a pulmonary consult.

Why Do I Need an Annual Physical?

An annual medical physical examination is very important for health protection. During a physical examination, the doctor usually begins with a vital check that includes blood pressure monitor ,temperature, and pulse rate, which may show that a patient has medical conditions such as high blood pressure that may result in stroke or heart attack in the future if not treated.

The next stage in the doctor visit involves history and examinations. Any skin lesions that may develop into cancer are detected. Any leg swelling suggesting a weak heart is noted, and a plan is made to prevent complications.

The doctor orders basic blood work, which may reveal a low blood count called anemia. This may indicate slow bleeding as well as early kidney problems, which if treated may prevent ending up in dialysis.

Keep your health maintenance appointments (mammogram, colonoscopy, Pap smear) or reschedule if you missed them. There is strong evidence that they help diagnose cancers at an early stage. Many patients appear and feel great, yet the body is hiding serious medical conditions until too late.

Ms. H. is a sixty-year-old female. She was enjoying good health until two months ago. She has been living a healthy lifestyle. She swims in the local recreational center. She only drinks wine socially on weekends. She smoked for ten years, but quit about seven years ago. She runs for thirty minutes daily.

She has not a seen a doctor for thirty years—since her college physical examination. She has never had a Pap smear, mammogram, or colonoscopy. She has no medical problems and takes no medication.

Over the last two months, she has been feeling weak. She is no longer able to run and gets tired after minimal activity. She lost twenty-five pounds unintentionally over the last month. Whenever she urinates, she sees large amounts of blood and blood clots. She is postmenopausal; her last menstrual period was ten years ago at the age of fifty.

What should she do?

A. Do not worry about it because stress and worry may cause hypertension.

B. She needs extra iron pills from over the counter to treat her anemia from blood loss. Nothing else.

C. She needs to see a doctor immediately because she might have cancer of the uterus or cervical cancer.

The correct answer is C. Vaginal bleeding after menopause is a concern for cancer of the uterus or cervical cancer. She needs an evaluation by a gynecologist as soon as possible. Options A and B are wrong. Delaying care because of assumptions is not a good idea.

The doctor needs enough information from you to write a note below (History and Physical), which is complete story of your medical condition. It is confidential.

Be honest. It will give the doctor the data to understand what is going on with your body to make the correct diagnosis to help you.

Secrets of Doctors Who Write Good History and Physical Reports

History of Present Illness

- Chief Complaints: chest pain, shortness of breath, slurred speech
- Demography: age, gender, race, occupation, and medical history
- Duration of Symptoms: months, weeks, days, hours
- Onset: sudden or gradual
- When: walking, sitting, eating, standing at home, at work, sleeping, playing
- Location of Symptoms: chest, abdomen, leg
- Quality: sharp, dull, pressure, tightness, clear food, non-bloody, size of a teaspoon

Intensity

- Scale of 1 to 10: moderate, severe, mild
- Intensity: constant or intermittent
- Frequency: last episode

- Radiation of Pain: left arm, shoulder, abdomen, back
- Aggravated: exertion, cough, movement, food
- Relief: rest, food, Tylenol, ibuprofen, over-the-counter medication, sleeping position
- Associated: fever, chills, nausea, vomiting, weight loss
- Trauma history: previous hospital admissions, results of investigations
- Previous episode: none, happened about years ago, was evaluated at a hospital

Review of System (at least ten systems must be completed)

- General: fever, chills
- Neurological: loss of consciousness, dizziness, extremity, weakness, weight loss, headache
- Ear, Nose, Throat: sore throat, runny nose, loss of hearing
- Eyes: blurry vision, double vision, jaundice, eye discharge
- Neck: stiffness, pain, swollen glands, jugular vein distention
- Cardiovascular System: chest pain, palpitations, orthopnea, PND
- Respiratory System: shortness of breath, leg swelling, exercise tolerance changed, cough not productive of green, whitish, scanty sputum
- Abdomen: rectal, nausea, vomiting, diarrhea, bloody stool

- Urinary: urinary frequency, leg swelling
- Musculoskeletal: joint pain, swelling, leg swelling
- Endocrinology: polyuria, polydisea, thyroid swelling
- Skin: rash, easy bruising
- Psychiatric: mood problem, depression
- Past Medical history: none, hypertension, diabetes, strokes, heart problems, kidney, atrial fibrillation, Coumadin use due to bleeding or compliance, fall risk

Surgical History

- Appendix: hernia, Caesarian section, gall bladder surgery, knee surgery, heart surgery
- Medication: dosage
- Allergies: none, penicillin
- Family history: heart attacks, strokes, kidney failure, seizures, depression
- Social History: tobacco usage
- Alcohol Usage: none, daily, socially
- Recreational Drug Use: none, Cocaine, heroin, marijuana
- Sexual Activity: married, multiple partners, condom use, STDs
- Living Situation: alone, with family, assisted living facility, skilled nursing facility

Physical Examination

- Vital Signs: Blood pressure, heart rate, breathing rate, temperature

- General: in respiratory distress, oriented in time, space, person, orthopnea, alert, depressed
- Head: Atraumatic , Normocephalic
- Eye. Normal reaction to light. Fundoscopy, abnormalities papillaedema
- Ear, Nose: clear, abnormal, discharge
- Mouth and Throat: lesions, good dentition, tonsils enlargement, erythema
- Neck: supple, JVD, carotid bruits, lymph nodes, thyroid enlargement
- External Edema: pulse, DTR, muscle group, cyanosis, clubbing, pale, joint deformity, tenderness,
- Heart: deformities, displaced PMI, Heaves, S1S2 regular, murmur, gallops
- Chest: unlabored breathing, auscultation, clear, crackles, rubs, rhonchi, wheezing stridor, percussion, dullness, tactile fremitus normal.
- Abdomen: surgical scars or skin abnormalities, bowel sounds present and normative in 4-quadrant on palpation mass, hepatomegaly, splenomegaly, Tenderness, rebound tenderness, CVA tenderness
- Guaiac: positive or negative
- Neuro Sensation: dull, sharp , C2, C 12, finger to nose, Babinski, memory, concentration, obeying command, able to draw clock at 5:20, hemiplegia
- Laboratory Investigation: complete blood count, chemistry panel

- Other investigations: EKG, tracing, reviewed, show, UA
- Chest: X-ray image reviewed, shown
- Old Discharge Summary: reviewed, shown
- Obtain More History from PCP
- Summarize to Patient in Simple Language.
- Allowed to Ask Questions
- Admitting Diagnosis Assessment
- Plan, Management
- Use protocol recent guidelines

Family Health Hints

Patients admitted to hospitals miss their family and loved ones. This is time to show that you care for them. Please visit them. Call them. Send cards. Keep dolls at the bedside. They will appreciate your love .

When It Is Time to Return Home

Sometimes our loved ones may need rehabilitation after long hospital stay because they may become weaker by staying long in the hospital. The level of care they need may be a burden to your family. For example, after hip fracture and surgery, they are not able to walk and require total care to eat or use the shower. The doctor may advise a short-term rehabilitation facility. They are properly equipped and have a trained staff for such care. Think about the options:

The patient was admitted for treatment of a condition that was diagnosed after he or she was presented to the emergency department with a cough.

His initial examination was consistent with the diagnosis of the treated condition.

During his hospital stay, he was admitted to ICU telemetry. In the medical ward, treatment included antibiotic medication via IV due to nausea, vomiting, and critical condition.

Consultations included pulmonary, cardiology, and recommended rehab.

The patient made remarkable improvement based on the management, He has good oral intake, no vomiting, is alert, and oriented to person, time, and place.

This discharge and follow-up plan has been discussed with the patient, family questions were answered, and instructions were understood.

Prepare Your Family
for Major Disaster

In a disaster or emergency, have supplies to last three days. Have enough medication refills for the elderly. Have water, food, touch lamps, batteries, essential documents, warm clothes, and a radio that uses batteries to communicate. Keep your vehicle gas tank near full at all times because you may need the car to stay warm and drive for hours to find safety.

Always think positively and forgive. It is good for your health.

Finally, when the doctor says you have no hope for cure, remember God is the greatest physician. The Almighty also knows when man needs eternal rest.

Medical References

American College of Medicine Medical Knowledge
Assessment Program (MKSAP series)
www.uptodate.com
Medstudy.com

Disclaimer

The medical information and forum opinion is provided
in good faith to help provide timely care to the sick and
needy but should not replace consultation with your
primary care physician or recent medical literature,
because medical information is dynamic and subject to
change with time.

About the Author

Onyechela Ogbonna, MD is a medical doctor with great clinical experience. He is board certified in internal medicine. He completed medical training at the Mount Sinai School of Medicine in Queens, New York.

His current clinical duty includes direct care to thousands of patients and supervising medical residents, students, nurses, physician assistants, and APRNs. He does medical consultations in the emergency department for management of complex conditions. He advises patients and their families on health-related issues.

He is a hospital physician based in Hartford Hospital, a major referral hospital in Hartford, Connecticut.